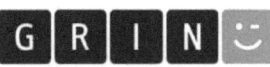

Bibliographic information published by the German National Library:

The German National Library lists this publication in the National Bibliography; detailed bibliographic data are available on the Internet at http://dnb.dnb.de .

Imprint:

Copyright © 2018 GRIN Verlag
Print and binding: Books on Demand GmbH, Norderstedt Germany
ISBN: 9783668700871

This book at GRIN:

https://www.grin.com/document/423819

Sagar Pamu

Drug interactions. How to recognise and how to manage them

GRIN Verlag

GRIN - Your knowledge has value

Since its foundation in 1998, GRIN has specialized in publishing academic texts by students, college teachers and other academics as e-book and printed book. The website www.grin.com is an ideal platform for presenting term papers, final papers, scientific essays, dissertations and specialist books.

Visit us on the internet:

http://www.grin.com/

http://www.facebook.com/grincom

http://www.twitter.com/grin_com

A Monograph of Drug Interactions

Author

Sagar Pamu

A Monograph of Drug Interactions

List of Contents

Introduction

Drug Interactions are an important cause of drug related problems and this includes significant morbidity and mortality. The ability to recognise and manage drug interactions is a crucial role of the pharmacist in optimising patient outcomes. An important skill is to be able to recognise clinically significant drug interactions and provide management advice to the patient and their doctor. This advice may include discussing dose alteration strategies or alternative non-interacting drug combinations.

Typically, interaction between drugs comes to mind (drug-drug interaction). However, interactions may also exist between drugs & foods (drug-food interactions), as well as drugs & herbs (drug-herb interactions). These may occur out of accidental misuse or due to lack of knowledge about the active ingredients involved in the relevant substances.

Drug-drug interactions cause hospitalizations attributed to drugs in the elderly. In most cases they are erroneously interpreted as patient deterioration because of illness, poor adherence to in treatment, or infection. In the United States 25% of ambulatory patients taking drug combinations were at risk for clinically important interactions [1].

Definition

A drug-drug interaction is defined as a pharmacokinetic or pharmacodynamic influence of drugs on each other, which may result in desired effects, in reduced efficacy and effectiveness or in increased toxicity.

A drug interaction is a situation in which a substance affects the activity of a drug, i.e. the effects are increased or decreased, or they produce a new effect that neither produces on its own.

Variability in pharmacokinetics (what the body does to the drug) and pharmacodynamics (what the drug does to the body) means that even clinically significant interactions are often unpredictable in the magnitude of their effect [2].

Epidemiology

- ❖ The true incidence is difficult to determine because data for drug-related hospital admissions do not separate out drug interactions, focus on ADRs.
- ❖ Patients receiving polypharmacy are at risk because 77% of HIV patients on protease inhibitors experience drug interactions.
- ❖ There are some patient categories that are at greater risk of experiencing a drug interaction. There are also some drugs, which tend to be involved in the more important clinically significant drug interactions
- ❖ High risk patients especially in the elderly are more prone to drug interactions, as they are more sensitive to some pharmacodynamic effects and also tend to be on more drugs. Patients on > 6 drugs have an 80% chance of a drug interaction. Many hospitals in patients are on 6 drugs or more.
- ❖ In the early 1990s, patients experienced serious cardiac toxicity after taking antihistamine or prokinetic drugs in combination with macrolide antibiotics or azole antifungals. It was identified that inhibiting cytochrome P450 (CYP450), 3A isoenzymes resulted in higher plasma

drug concentrations. Subsequently, terfenadine, astemizole, and cisapride were withdrawn from the marketplace, in part because of safety concerns about drug interactions.

❖ High risk drugs include with a narrow therapeutic index, i.e. a relatively small change in the plasma concentration can cause drug toxicity or sub therapeutic effect. Thus, a pharmacokinetic interaction which changes the plasma concentration (up or down) will cause a change in effect.

❖ Warfarin and the other oral anticoagulants fall in to a special high-risk category. The clinical effect of warfarin is measured from the prothrombin time or INR and the dose is titrated to provide a sufficient degree of anticoagulation without causing bleeding. Drugs or agents which change the pharmacokinetics of warfarin can have a dramatic clinical effect. Agents that change the supply or synthesis of vitamin K can also alter the pharmacodynamic effect of warfarin.

❖ Other drug classes with important interactions include antidepressants, antiarrhythmics, antipsychotics, hypoglycaemic agents. Also note that the commonly used drugs cimetidine and erythromycin are potent enzyme inhibitors.

❖ Some drugs with a low therapeutic index Lithium, Digoxin, Carbamazepine, Cyclosporin Phenytoin, Phenobarbitone, Theophylline, (Aminophylline) Warfarin[3].

How do drug interactions occur? [4]

There are several mechanisms by which drugs interact with other drugs, food, and other substances. An interaction can result when there is an increase or decrease in: the absorption of a drug into the body; distribution of the drug within the body; alterations made to the drug by the body (metabolism); and elimination of the drug from the body. One notable system involved in metabolic drug interactions is the enzyme system comprising the cytochrome P450 oxidizes. This system may be affected by either enzyme induction or enzyme inhibition.

Most of the important drug interactions result from a change in the absorption, metabolism, or elimination of a drug. Drug interactions also may occur when two drugs that have similar (additive) effects or opposite (cancelling) effects on the body are administered together. For example, there may be major sedation when two drugs that has sedation as side effects are given, such as, narcotics and antihistamines.

Another source of drug interactions occurs when one drug alters the concentration of a substance that is normally present in the body. The alteration of this substance reduces or enhances the effect of another drug that is being taken. The drug interaction between warfarin (Coumadin) and vitamin K-containing products is a good example of this type of interaction. Warfarin acts by reducing the concentration of the active form of vitamin K in the body. Therefore, when vitamin K is taken, it reduces the effect of warfarin.

Reasons for increased drug interactions

- Drug abuse and misuse.

- Patients consult several physicians.

- Concurrent use of prescription and non-prescription drugs.

- Patient non-compliance.

- Drug potency.

The remaining drug interactions are in formidable challenge for several reasons. The science of drug interactions is complex and constantly evolving, the patient's medication list is often a moving target with prescription and non-prescription elements, and dozens of new drugs arrive at our pharmacies each year, often with incompletely characterized drug interaction profiles. The risk of harm due to drug interactions can be lessened by awareness of these principles, thoughtful prescribing habits and judicious monitoring when new drugs are added to regimens.

Medicines are often used concomitantly with other drugs, and some degree of drug interaction occurs with concomitant use. Although only a small proportion of this interaction is clinically significant, it sometimes causes serious adverse reactions. For example, drug interactions, particularly with drugs having a narrow therapeutic range, may have serious adverse consequences. Therefore, in the evaluation and clinical application of drugs, appropriate efforts should be made to predict the nature and degree of drug interactions so that patients will not be adversely affected. Humans are genetically diverse, and disease states are likewise diverse. It should, therefore, be kept in mind that drug interactions might readily cause clinically significant changes in blood drug levels (concentration in whole blood, plasma, or serum) in patients having pharmacokinetic parameters markedly deviating from those of the standard population. Drug interactions may occur after administration by any route.

A multiplicity of outcomes is possible when people use drugs. Most commonly the patient benefits from drug therapy; however, adverse events, ranging from minor side effects to death, may occur. One of the consequences of multiple drug use is the risk of one drug influencing the activity, the availability or the effect of a second drug. Drugs have most likely been used in combinations to potentiate their intended effects. Indeed, it may be favourable to use a combination of drugs if that combination is well documented to enhance the effect or to reduce adverse effects. However, physicians may advertently prescribe improper combinations that result in less effect or more adverse drug reactions [1].

Drug-drug interactions can lead to severe side effects and have resulted in early termination of development of drugs, refusal of approval, severe prescribing restrictions and withdrawal of drugs from the market. Whether a given magnitude of effect of an interacting inhibitory drug (i.e., Precipitant drug) on plasma levels of a recipient drug (i.e., Object drug) which results in an increased risk of adverse events depends to a great extent on the therapeutic index of the recipient drug. Even small pharmacokinetic interactions can result in significant pharmacodynamic adverse effects for drugs of a narrow therapeutic index. However, small to moderate pharmacokinetic interactions may not necessarily result in detectable and clinically significant consequences for drugs of a wider therapeutic index. Many physicians and other health care providers have only a rudimentary knowledge regarding drug-drug interactions.

With the seemingly constant flow of new therapeutic agents and new treatment indications for existing medications, polypharmacy is increasingly common. Many drug interactions are avoidable, but those that are not require awareness of the interaction to allow for proper management and appropriate dosage adjustments. The issue of drug interactions is bound to come up. It is therefore prudent to learn about such interactions so they can be effectively managed. Intelligent choices with respect to medication combinations can be made, and doses can be adjusted to keep patients in safe therapeutic zones.

An interaction is said to occur when the effects of one drug are changed by the presence of another drug, food, drink or by some environmental chemical agent. The outcome can be harmful if the interactions cause an increase in the toxicity of the drug. A reduction in efficacy due to an interaction can sometimes be just as harmful as an increase in toxicity (i.e. when antibiotics are combined with ions or antacids, the effects of these antibiotics can be reduced or even abolished in the gut).

Drug interactions may make a drug less effective, cause unexpected side effects or increase the action of a particular drug. Drug interactions fall into three broad categories,

Drug – drug interactions

Drug – food interactions

Drug – condition interactions

Drug – drug interactions occur when the administration of a drug results in decreased effectiveness or increased toxicity of other drugs that are also being taken (e.g., Heparin when combined with aspirin increases risk of bleeding).

Drug – food interactions occur when the effectiveness of the drug is decreased or the toxicity increased because of its interaction with foods (e.g.,

Tetracycline when taken with milk or calcium rich foods it decreases the effect of tetracycline).

Drug – condition interactions may occur when an existing medical condition makes certain drug potentially harmful (e.g., Tobramycin in combination with frusemide in renal failure patient's worse the condition by increasing the nephrotoxicity).

Factors of Drug Interaction

There are multiple factors that can influence the outcome of a drug interaction. These factors are based on the properties of the object drug and the precipitating drug.

Object Drugs

- Those which have low therapeutic index (e.g., Digoxin)
- Those which have a steep dose-response curve (e.g., aminoglycoside antibiotics.)

Precipitant Drugs

- Those which are highly protein bound (e.g., Aspirin), and therefore likely to displace   object drugs from protein binding sites.
- Those which stimulate (e.g., rifampicin) or inhibit (e.g., cimetidine) the metabolism of other drugs.
- Those which affect renal function (e.g., Probenecid) and alter the renal clearance of object drug.

Drug interactions refer to the interference of a drug in the action of another drug or the interference of food or nutrient in the action of drugs. It is estimated that interactions occur in 3 to 5% of patients receiving four drugs, and when 10 to 20 drugs are used, this rate reaches 20%.

Drug interactions may produce beneficial or undesirable. The beneficial effects are those whose purpose is to treat concomitant diseases, enhancing the effectiveness, reducing adverse effects and allowing to reduce the dose, while the undesirable effects may reduce the drug effectiveness, and may produce adverse and even toxic effects in the body, besides increased treatment cost.

The undesirable interactions may be subdivided into **severe** interactions, which may produce a risk to life or permanent damages, **moderate** interactions, which require additional treatment, and **mild** interactions, which do not affect significantly the therapy effect [2].

Types of Drug Interactions

The drug interactions are divided into 3 types they are pharmaceutical drug interaction, pharmacokinetic drug interaction and, pharmacodynamics drug interaction.

Pharmaceutical Drug Interactions

Pharmaceutical interactions can be a pharmacodynamic or pharmacokinetic. Some drug interactions are due to a combination of mechanisms.

These interactions are due to competition at receptor sites or activity of the interacting drugs on the same physiological system. There is no change in the plasma concentrations of interacting drugs.

Pharmaceutical drug interaction is known as drug incompatibilities, occur before the drug administration in the body, when two or more of them are mixed in the syringe or other recipient, and are evidenced by organoleptic alterations, reduced or interrupted activity of one or both drugs or formation of a new compound.

- Drugs with opposing pharmacological actions acting on the same receptor(**antagonist**). E.g. salbutamol (a beta-2 agonist) with metoprolol (a beta-2 antagonist).

- Drugs with a similar pharmacological action may have an additive effect (**additive/synergistic**). E.g. Fluoxetine (an SSRI) with clomipramine (a tricyclic antidepressant with serotonergic activity) can cause serotonin syndrome in some patients.

- Fluid or electrolyte imbalance. Drugs with a similar pharmacological action may have an additive effect. E.g. diuretics that cause hypokalaemia can increase the toxicity of digoxin.

- NSAID's can reduce the effectiveness of antihypertensive by causing salt and water retention(**indirect interaction**)

E.g. Fluoxetine (an SSRI) with clomipramine (a tricycles antidepressant with serotonergic activity) can cause serotonin syndrome in some patients.

Pharmacokinetic Drug Interactions

Pharmacokinetic is known as "what the body does to the drug". In this pharmacokinetic one drug can alter the concentration of other drug.

Pharmacokinetic interaction occurs during the process of drug absorption, distribution, biotransformation and excretion, resulting in increased or reduced plasmatic concentration and consequently alteration to the pharmacological effect.

➢ **Absorption**

Drugs that are orally administered are generally absorbed from the gastrointestinal (GI) tract into the systemic circulation. There is a high probability for drug interactions to occur during their movement through the GI tract. Drug absorption occurs by either passive or active transport, with most drugs being absorbed by passive transport. This process involves diffusion of a drug from areas with a high drug concentration to regions with lower concentrations. Active transport involves the movement of drugs (i.e., ions and water-soluble molecules) against a concentration gradient (i.e., from regions of low concentration to areas of high concentration) and therefore requires an energy source. Drug absorption that occurs by active transport is usually more rapid than that which occurs by passive diffusion. The non-ionized form of a drug is lipid soluble and readily diffuses across the cell membrane, while the ionized form of the drug is lipid insoluble and non-diffusible. Under normal physiologic conditions, drug absorption can be slightly delayed, but the extent of absorption is usually complete. In some instances, a drug's dosage form may contribute to the interaction.

For example, most of the Theophylline products are recommended to be taken with food to avoid GI upset. However, if the drug product-Theophylline is taken without food, the timed-release mechanism of this dosage form is disrupted and it becomes an immediate-release product, leading to significantly increased Theophylline absorption and potentially toxic peak serum levels

Drug Interactions Involving Altered Absorption-

When the absorption rate of a drug is altered, clinically significant drug interactions are more likely to occur, especially when the drug has a short half-life or it requires a rapid peak plasma drug level to achieve a therapeutic effect. Drug interactions involving a drug's GI absorption generally result in a decrease rather than an increase in drug absorption. The mechanisms of action for these interactions include:

1) Altered gastrointestinal pH-values;

2) The formation of insoluble complexes or chelated compounds;

3) Drugs being bound to bile acid sequestrant (BAS) drugs;

4) Altered GI function (acceleration or slowing of gastric emptying, change in vascular or permeability of GI mucosa, or mucosal damage of the gut wall); and

5) Altered intestinal blood flow.

Of these possible mechanisms of action, most clinically significant drug interactions result from the formation of insoluble complexes, or chelates, and when drugs are bound to resins that bind bile acids. Although it is certainly possible, few clinically significant drug interactions occur as a result of changes in intestinal blood flow or from changes in gastric motility. However, there are some striking drug interactions with drugs that alter GI tract pH, i.e., antacids that lead to a significant decrease in drug bioavailability.

Drug interactions between Fluoroquinolones antibiotics (e.g., Ciprofloxacin, Enoxacin, Levofloxacin, Lomefloxacin, Norfloxacin, and Sparfloxacin) and divalent or trivalent ions (i.e., Calcium, Magnesium, and Aluminum ions from antacids and other drug products) can lead to a significant decrease in GI absorption, bioavailability and therapeutic effects. Also, these interactions can severely diminish the activity of Fluoroquinolones antibiotics. The effects of these interactions can be significantly reduced by administering antacid doses several hours before or after giving the Fluoroquinolone drug. If an antacid is absolutely required, adjunctive therapy, such as an H2 receptor antagonist or a proton pump inhibitor, may be used to replace the antacid in the treatment of peptic ulcer disease. When patients use antacid products, particularly

Magnesium Aluminum hydroxide antacids, they should be encouraged to avoid taking the antacid within two hours after a Fluoroquinolone dose or in, the six hours prior to the next antimicrobial dose. Antacid products containing Calcium or Magnesium, Zinc, and Iron supplements produce a less significant effect, but they should still be separated from Quinolone administration. Similarly, the drug Sucralfate also interacts with a number of Fluoroquinolones in this manner, and it is recommended that Ciprofloxacin be administered several hours before or six hours after a Sucralfate dose. Since Sucralfate is generally administered four times daily, one potential solution to this problem is to discontinue using Sucralfate Products while taking Fluoroquinolone antibiotics.

> ### Distribution

After a drug is absorbed into the systemic circulation, it is transported to target sites where it reacts with various body tissues and/or receptors. While transversing the blood, drugs can bind to various blood components, especially the protein albumin. Lipid-soluble drugs have a high affinity for adipose tissue, which is where these drugs are stored. The relatively low blood flow to fat tissue makes it as reservoir for lipid-soluble drugs. This drug depot prolongs the effects of the drugs. Drugs that are highly lipid soluble include Phenothiazines, Benzodiazepines and Barbiturates. A number of acidic drugs have an affinity to bind blood sites on proteins, particularly albumin. Plasma protein binding (PPB) of drugs is expressed as a percent, which represents the percent of total drug that is bound.

The portion of drug that binds to albumin is pharmacologically inactive, while the unbound portion of drug, or the free fraction, is pharmacologically active. When two or more highly protein-bound drugs are administered concurrently, competitive binding for the same site may result in displacement of one of the drugs from protein binding, increasing the amount of free drug in the blood. When one drug is displaced from its binding sites on plasma proteins by another drug, there is a transient increase in free drug that is distributed through various tissues. Patients with hypoalbuminemia will have free drug or active drug available.

Drugs most likely to be involved in clinically significant interactions include:

   (1) Highly protein bound (~90% or greater),

   (2) Bound in tissues,

   (3) Small volume of distribution (V d),

   (4) Low hepatic extraction ratio,

   (5) Narrow therapeutic index,

   (6) Rapid onset of action, or

   (7) Administered intravenously.

Drugs with the highest capability to displace other drugs from protein binding sites include Salicylic acid, Phenylbutazone, Sulphonamides, and Nonsteroidal anti-inflammatory drugs (NSAIDs). Highly protein-bound drugs can interact with drugs like Warfarin. They increase its pharmacologic effects by displacing it from protein binding sites and altering its metabolism. Some drugs that are highly protein bound also have the ability to inhibit or induce enzymatic metabolic activity. Therefore, multiple mechanisms for the interaction are possible. For example, Warfarin interacts with Suifamethoxazole-trimethoprim, resulting in an increased anticoagulant effect.

Receptor Binding of Drugs:

A small number of clinically significant drug interactions are caused when a drug is displaced from its receptor sites by another drug. For example, Guanidine can displace Digoxin from binding sites in skeletal muscle, increasing the serum concentration of Digoxin (other mechanism may also be involved) and possibly producing Digoxin toxicity. Similarly, Propranolol can precipitate an asthmatic attack because as a nonselective beta-blocker it can displace Terbutaline, a beta agonist, from beta- - 2 receptors.

➢ Metabolism

To produce a systemic physiologic effect in the body, most drugs must reach receptor sites, which mean they must be able to cross lipid plasma membranes. To accomplish this task, drugs must be somewhat lipid soluble. One role of metabolism is to convert active lipid-soluble compounds to inactive water-soluble substances that can be excreted, primarily by the kidneys. Drugs may go through two different metabolic processes, Phase I and Phase II metabolism.

In Phase I metabolism, hepatic microsomal enzymes contained in the endothelium of liver cells first oxidize, demethylate,. hydrolyze, etc., drugs to render them more water soluble. In Phase II large water soluble substances (e.g., Glucuronic acid, Sulphate) are attached to the drug to form inactive or significantly less active, water-soluble metabolites. Compounds may circulate through one or both phases multiple times until the water-soluble characteristic is present. More clinically significant drug interactions are caused by Phase I hepatic microsomal enzymes rather than by Phase II metabolism. Most drug metabolism takes place in the liver, but other organs, such as the kidneys, lungs and intestinal tract are also involved. Drugs identified as high extraction drugs are almost entirely metabolized during the first pass through the liver. In general, high-extraction ratio drugs are less affected by interactions than low-extraction drugs.

These drugs usually have a short half-life, and their metabolites are usually inactive. However, the lower the therapeutic index of a drug, the more serious the potential consequences of drug interactions affecting metabolism. In some instances, a drug interaction may result from the sequence in which drugs are administered. For example, a drug interaction is unlikely to occur when anticoagulant therapy with Warfarin is initiated in a patient stabilized on

Thyroid replacement therapy. However, when a patient already receiving oral anticoagulant [3].

High-Risk Patients and Drug Interactions

The magnitude of the drug interactions problem increases significantly in certain patient populations and as the number of medications taken each day increases. Drug interactions that may be of minor clinical significance in patients with less severe forms of a disease can cause significant exacerbation of the clinical condition in patients with more severe forms of the disease. Patient populations at high risk include the elderly, critical care patients, and patients undergoing complicated surgical procedures. The elderly population is at high risk because of the number of medications consumed, complicated drug regimens, and clinical states often presented. About 80% of elderly patients routinely take prescription and non-prescription medications concurrently. Some patients may see multiple physicians for acute and chronic conditions, as well as obtain medication from more than one community pharmacy or mail-order Pharmacy.

Conditions that Place Patients at High Risk for Drug Interactions

1. High risk associated with the severity of disease state being treated Aplastic anaemia, Asthma, Cardiac arrhythmia, Critical care/intensive Care patients, Diabetes, Epilepsy, Hepatic disease, Hypothyroid.

2. High risk associated with drug interaction potential of related therapy.Autoimmune disease, cardiovascular gastrointestinal Infection, Psychiatric disease, Respiratory disorders, Seizure disorders.

Drugs with Narrow Therapeutic Index

Aminoglycoside antibiotics (Gentamicin, Tobramycin), Anti coagulants (Warfarin, Heparins), Aspirin, Carbamazepine, Conjugated estrogens, Cyclosporine, Digoxin, Esterified estrogens, Hypoglycemic Agents,

Levothyroxine sodium, Lithium, Phenytoin, Procainamide, Quinidine sulfate/gluconate. Drugs identified as having a high risk of being involved in a clinically significant drug interaction frequently have a narrow therapeutic index, a very steep dose-response curve or potent pharmacologic effects. A toxic dose of these drugs may be only slightly above the therapeutic dose. A slight increase in the dose may produce a large increase in serum drug levels and clinical effect. Conversely, a slight decrease in the plasma level of drugs with a steep dose response curve may result in a significant loss of therapeutic effect. Examples of such drugs include Corticosteroids, Carbamazepine, Quinidine, Oral contraceptives, and Rifampicin. Patients receiving drugs with a narrow therapeutic index should be monitored closely for possible clinically significant drug interactions.

> ## Elimination

Drug interactions that occur at the level of excretion may involve one or more of the following:

(1) Glomerular filtrations,

(2) Active secretion or passive reabsorption in the renal tubular system, or

(3) Competition of drugs for the same active transport system.

Drugs with the ability to increase or decrease golmerular filtration by altering the renal blood flow may influence the rate of excretion of other drugs or their active or inactive metabolites. For drugs with narrow therapeutic reactions, increasing their renal clearance reduces their plasma steady – state concentrations, whereas interference with the renal excretion mechanisms will increase their circulating level and may result in toxic drug levels. Drug interactions can occur when changes in urinary pH alter the excretion of weakly acidic or weakly basic drugs by affecting their extent of ionization. This consequently affects their reabsorption from the lumen of renal tubules.

For example, acidifying urine with Ascorbic acid or other drugs can increase serum Phenobarbital levels, and alkalizing urine with antacids can decrease serum salicylate (salicylic acid) levels. Other drug interactions can occur in the kidneys when one drug's normal renal excretion, involving active transport in the renal tubules, modified by another drug. For example, when the drug probenecid is co administered with certain antibiotics (i.e. Penicillin, Ampicillin, or Amoxicillin) the two drugs compacts for excretion. In this instance, drug excretion favours probenecid. The antibiotic is retained and reabsorbed, leading to elevated and prolonged serum levels of the antibiotic. Often, clinicians use this interaction to their advantage, to achieve higher and prolonged antibiotic blood level in patients using lower doses of the antibiotic.

Another example of this reaction occurs with the co – administration of Quinidine and Digoxin. In this situation, drug excretion through the kidneys favours Quinidine and leads to increased blood levels of Digoxin. When diuretics or low- salt diets decrease the amount of sodium present, sodium and Lithium compete for excretions via the kidneys in patients taking Lithium. In this situation, Lithium will be excreted while sodium will be retained. The result is an increased excretion of Lithium and decrease serum drug levels

Pharmacodynamic Drug Interactions

Pharmacodynamic is known as "what the drug does to the body". It is related to the drug effects in the body. In this pharmacodynamic one drug modulates the effect of other drug i.e., additive, synergistic or antagonistic.

Regarding the treatment of a drug interaction occurrence that may be harmful to the patient, the health professional should: avoid complex therapeutic systems, adopt alternative measures, provide instructions on the correct interval between drug administrations, determine the probability of important interaction occurrences and monitor the patient. With the high number of reports on new drug interactions, it has been difficult for health professionals to keep constantly updated. Today, computer systems are used to verify the risk of potential drug interactions, thus preventing the utilization of drugs that cause important and harmful interactions and reducing the patient's exposure to them.

It was found in large surveys that approximately 60% of inpatients in general medical wards were at risk of drug interactions, and studies conducted in hospital emergency departments found that from 16% to 47% of inpatients were at risk of drug interactions.

Onset of Drug interactions are of 3 types.

❖ **Rapid:** Onset of clinical conflict or adverse effects expected within 24 hours of drug administration.

❖ **Delayed:** Onset of clinical conflict or adverse effects not expected to appear within the first 24 hours following drug administration.

❖ **Unspecified:** Not reported in the literature.

Drug-drug interaction should be suspected anytime a new or an unexpected effect occurs and complicates the clinical management of a patient in a setting where the patient is receiving at least 2 interacting drugs.

Drug-drug interactions cause hospitalizations attributed to drugs in the elderly. In most cases they are erroneously interpreted as patient deterioration because of illness, poor adherence to prescribed treatment, or infection. In the

United States 25% of ambulatory patients taking drug combinations were at risk for clinically important interactions.

Drug–drug interactions in the field of infectious diseases continue to expand as new drugs are approved, metabolic enzymes and transporters are identified, and recommendations for co administration of drugs are revised. Fluoroquinolones are used routinely in outpatients, given their excellent oral bioavailability and safety profile. Since fluoroquinolones have concentration-dependent pharmacodynamics, implying that reductions in maximium concentration (Cmax) and AUC values can lead to therapeutic failure [4].

Antibiotics are prescribed for longer durations than are other agents routinely administered. For example, local anaesthetics and sedatives usually are given in a single course of therapy, whereas in most patients analgesics are taken for a few days on an as needed basis. The typical antibiotic regimen for an infection is of a five- to 10-day duration on an around-the-clock schedule. This more chronic dosing sets the stage for some rather serious and potentially life-threatening drug interactions involving antimicrobial agents which inhibit the gut wall and liver cytochrome P-450 system with a host of other drugs that use the same metabolic pathway.

It is apparent that the fluoroquinolones represent an important advancement in infectious disease therapy. However, like other antimicrobial compounds, they are not without side effects. An understanding and appreciation of fluoroquinolone-drug interactions is essential for their optimal clinical use. Many questions concerning the potential of the fluoroquinolones with regard to drug interactions still remain. In addition, the majority of research on fluoroquinolone-drug interactions has been done in the research centre environment using normal, healthy adult volunteers. The clinical significance of fluoroquinolone-drug interactions needs to be based upon observations in various patient populations, where feasible. Many of the aforementioned interactions could be influenced by race, dosage regimen design, smoking status of the patient, diet composition, and underlying organ function. As the development of the fluoroquinolones continues, so does the appreciation that many compounds interact with these agents. There is an increase in the investigation of whether or not one or another compound interacts with a particular fluoroquinolone. The interaction of fluoroquinolones with theophylline has been widely studied. Indeed, many of the fluoroquinolones inhibit the metabolism of theophylline to such an extent that toxicity occurs.

Fluoroquinolones- norfloxacin, ciprofloxacin, and pefloxacin have also been shown to reduce the total body clearance of theophylline to varying degrees quinolones can interact with theophylline such that a reduction in theophylline dosage or removal of the quinolone from a patient's drug therapy regimen is necessary to prevent markedly elevated theophylline plasma concentrations from occurring.

Antibiotics that are commonly prescribed in the emergency department (ED) may lead to serious and even fatal interactions with warfarin and digoxin. Ciprofloxacin and trimethoprim-sulfamethoxazole may enhance the anticoagulant effect of warfarin. Clarithromycin, erythromycin, and tetracycline have been shown to increase digoxin levels by altering the gut flora that is important in digoxin metabolism. Commonly prescribed antibiotics, including microlides (erythromycin, azithromycin, and clarithromycin) and quinolones (ciprofloxacin and levofloxacin), may be associated with QT prolongation. These antibiotics should be used with particular caution in patients on other medications that may prolong the QT interval, such as class IA antiarrhythmics (quinidine, disopyramide, and procainamide) and class III antiarrhythmics (sotalol and amiodarone) [3].

Older people use many medicines because they suffer from more chronic conditions that need treatment by means of pharmacotherapy. Because of the higher number of medicines used and decline in hepatic and renal function, older patients are more prone to problems caused by these medicines. However, older people are more prone to adverse drug reactions, resulting from age-related factors such as changes in drug distribution, metabolism and excretion, and in receptor sensitivity as well as from drug–drug interactions and drug–disease interactions caused by prescribing of multiple drugs.

In other words, prescribing in older patients involves balancing conflicting demands, and the benefit risk ratio should be considered when deciding whether to initiate pharmacotherapy. Therefore, it is important to review pharmacotherapy concerning older patients in a reliable way [4].

Guidelines for Drug Interactions

It is not enough for the health care provider to be informed that two drugs may interact. It is also important to have information on measures that can be taken to reduce the likelihood of an adverse outcome.

Management options include:

❖ Avoiding the combination entirely. For some drug interactions, the risk always outweighs the benefit, and the combination should be avoided. Because drug classes are usually heterogeneous with regard to drug interactions (as described above) one can often select a non-interacting alternative for either the object drug or the precipitant drug.

❖ Adjusting the dose of the object drug. Sometimes, it is possible to give the two interacting drugs safely [5].

❖ Spacing dosing times to avoid the interaction. For some drug interactions involving binding in the gastrointestinal tract, to avoid the interaction one can give the object drug at least two hours before or four hours after the precipitant drug. In this way the object drug can be absorbed into the circulation before the precipitant drug appears.

❖ Monitoring for early detection. In some cases, when it is necessary to administer interacting drug combinations, the interaction can be managed through close laboratory or clinical monitoring for evidence of the interaction. In this way the appropriate dosage changes can be made, or the drugs discontinued if necessary.

❖ Monitoring of potential drug interactions may improve the quality of prescribing and dispensing and it might form a basis for education focused on appropriate prescribing [6].

The Swiss cheese model for Identifying Steps to Prevent Drug Interactions [7, 8]

'The Swiss cheese model of accident causation' by James Reason, a British psychologist, was adapted by Hansten and Horn to the problem of drug interactions which systematically illustrates the avoidance/occurrence of an adverse drug reaction caused by a drug interaction (Figure 1). Because adverse drug reactions resulting from drug interactions are almost completely preventable it is important to identify the steps at which that prevention can take place. Perfect systems do not exist. The holes in the Swiss cheese represent gaps in the defences.

Figure No: 1 Swiss cheese model for identifying steps to prevent drug

interactions

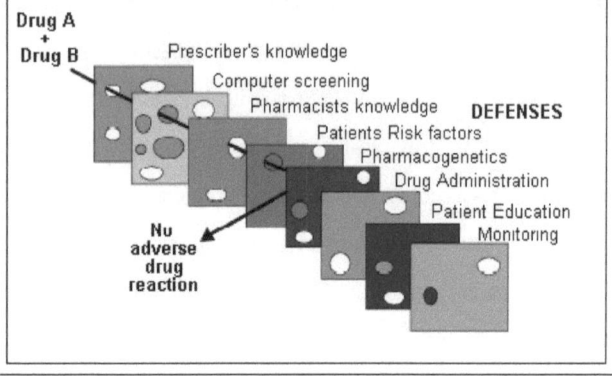

Drug interaction information sources [9, 10]

In the past 40 years more than 20000 journal articles on drug interactions have been published. This flood of information has overwhelmed even the most dedicated and compulsive of health care providers. No one can possibly memorise all the potential drug interactions that have been identified to date, and new interacting drug pairs are identified every month. To cope with this task drug interaction compendia in the form of books, computer or personal digital assistant (PDA) software or online databases are offered to health care providers. Studies revealing the prevalence of potential drug interactions often refer the US-database by Thompson Micromedex (TM) or the British Stockley's drug interactions, which can be considered as standard referenced information sources. Simply knowing that two drugs may interact does not provide enough information for the health care provider. It is also important to have information on measures that can be taken to reduce the likelihood of an adverse outcome. Therefore, drug interaction monographs have to contain information about the potential adverse effect, the rating of severity of the potential adverse event, and suggestions for the clinical management including dose-adjustment, sequential dosing time, alternative therapies, monitoring or patient related risk factors.

Evaluation of drug interactions:

There are about more than 6000 drugs available worldwide, along with traditional medicines and herbal remedies that can potentially interact. It is important to use pharmacological knowledge together with the medical literature to evaluate a potential drug interaction. Information is available from a wide range of sources such as in vitro and animal studies, case reports, clinical trials, review papers, handbooks, and monographs in books, paragraphs in product data sheets or on the World Wide Web. It is important that pharmacist is familiar with and use this information appropriately.

1. In vitro and animal data

Information from in vitro studies and animal experiments is helpful in identifying mechanisms for a drug interaction. Animal and invitro information cannot reliably predict that an interaction will occur in humans, as human pharmacodynamic process and physiology are not represented [11].

2. Case Reports

Interactions are often first identified as case reports or letters published in medical journals or reported to a pharmacovigilance program. The reliability of information in letters and case reports requires careful evaluation, as letter sections do not undergo peer review in most journals. Case reports are a useful source for identifying interactions between infrequently used drug combinations for rarely occurring interactions.

3. Clinical Trials

Clinical trials provide the most reliable evidence to support an interaction though controlling for extraneous factors (that could also explain the effect of drug interaction), and by providing a statistical estimation for the effect arising by chance [12].

4. Review, Monographs and Hand books

Review on drug interactions often appears in the pharmacy literature, for example recent series have been published in the pharmaceutical journal (UK) and annals of Pharmacotherapy. The purpose of these articles is education, although some reviews will provide reliable lists for interaction screening. Some useful books which contain complications of drug interactions, for example Stockley IH Drug Interactions is a standard book that provides details about drug interactions. It is also very important to check for more recently published information in the medical literature especially for recently introduced medicines and infrequent interactions or rarely used drug combinations [13].

5. Tables, Charts and Data sheets

Quick reference source for screening known drug interactions come in a variety of forms, of which the British National Formulary (BNF) tables is one of the better known. There are also wall or pocket sized charts and interaction warnings with dispensing computer programs that can assist rapid identification of an interaction. Product data sheets can provide useful information provided they have undergone independent review.

6. Interaction Websites

There is an increasing number of websites, which contain information on drug interactions. Some sites cover specific classes of drugs or conditions, for example, herbal medicines or medicines used to treat HIV/AIDS. Some sites like Dave Flockhart's Cytochrome P450 isoenzyme site is accurate and current.

This site is particularly useful for screening for suspected metabolic interactions, but it does predict clinical relevance and excludes many metabolized drugs for which the isoenzyme system involved have not been identified [14].

BIBLIOGRAPHY

1. Stockley IH. Drug interactions. In: A source book of adverse interactions, their mechanisms, clinical importance and management. 5th ed. London: Pharmaceutical Press; 1999. 1-14

2. Tipnis HP, Amrita B. Clinical Pharmacy. 1st ed. India: Career Publications; 2003

3. Cristiano Moura, Francisco Acurcio, Najara Belo. Drug-Drug Interactions Associated with Length of Stay and Cost of Hospitalization. J Pharm Pharmaceut Sci (www.cspsCanada.org), 2009 12(3), 266 – 272.

4. Daniel C. Malone, Jacob Abarca, Philip D. Hansten, Amy J. Grizzle. Identification of Serious Drug-Drug Interactions: Results of the Partnership to Prevent Drug-Drug Interactions. Journal of the American Pharmaceutical Association, mjapha.org March 2004 Vol. 44, No. 2, 142-152.

5. Hansten PD. Drug interaction management. Pharm World Sci 2003; 25(3): 94–97.

6. Indermitte J, Erba L, Beutler M, Bruppacher, Haefeli WE, Hersberger KE. Management of Potential Drug Interactions in community pharmacies. J Clin Phar Ther 2006 Jan 8; 32: 132-42.

7. Astrand E, Astrand B, Antonov K, Petersson G. Potential drug interactions during a three decade study period: a cross sectional study of a prescription register. Eur J clin Pharmacol 2007; 63(9): 851-9.

8. Bjornsson TD, Callaghan JT, Einolf HJ, Fischer V, Gan L, Grimm S et al. The conduct of in vitro and in vivo drug-drug interaction studies: a PhRMA perspective. J Clin Pharmacol 2003; 43: 443-469.

9. Alfaro CL, Piscitelli SC. Drug interactions. In:Atkinson AJ, Daniels CE, Dedrick RL, Grudyinllas CU, Markey SP, editors. Principles of clinical pharmacology San Diego, USA: Academic press; 2001.P.167- 80

10. Martinbiancho J, Zuckermann J, Dos Santos L, Silva MM. Profile of drug interactions in hospitalized children. J Pharmacy Practice 2007; 5(4): 157-161.

11. Riechelmann RP, Tannock IF, Wang L, Saad ED, Taback NA, Krzyzanowska MK. Potential Drug Interactions and Duplicate Prescriptions Among Cancer Patients. JNCI 2007; 99(8): 592-600.

12. Cruciol-Souza JM, Thomson JC. A pharmacoepidemiologic study of drug interactions in a brazilian teaching hospital. Clinics 2006; 61(6): 515-20.

13. Doubova SV, Reyes-Morales H, Torres-Arreola LP, Suárez- Ortega M. Potential drug-drug and drug-disease interactions in prescriptions for ambulatory patients over 50 years of age in family medicine clinics in Mexico City. BMC Health Services Research 2007; 147(7): 1-8.

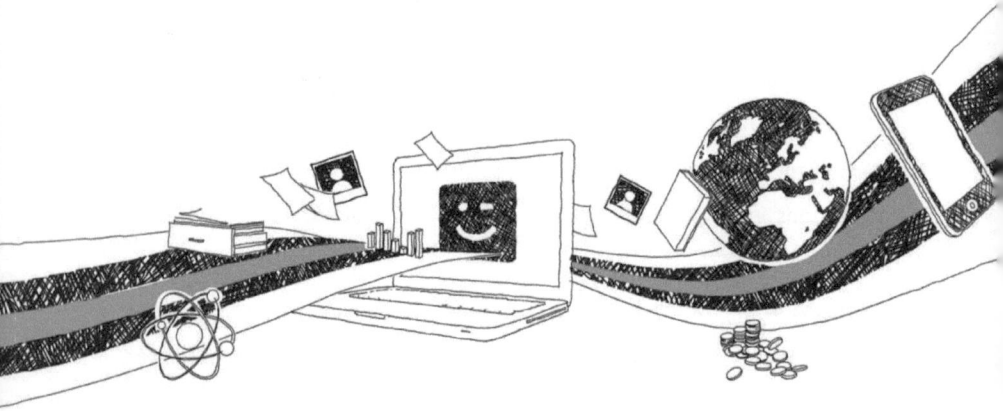
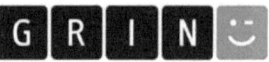